Ketogenic Diet

Weight Loss Mistakes to Stop

The information herein is offered for informational purposes solely, and is universal as so. The presentation of the information is without contract or any type of guarantee assurance.

The trademarks that are used are without any consent, and the publication of the trademark is without permission or backing by the trademark owner. All trademarks and brands within this book are for clarifying purposes only and are the owned by the owners themselves, not affiliated with this document.

Table of Contents

Introduction

Dieting is a tough path to follow. Most of us have all been there. We start our diet with bright, positive thoughts for our future. We dream of being healthy, and losing this excess weight that we like to think is making us miserable. As soon as we lose this weight, we will be happy, right? The next thing you know, you're a week into your diet, and you've never been more miserable in your life. Even when you think you're making all the right choices, you're not losing the weight. What are you doing wrong?

The truth is: it could be nothing, or it could be something. The fact of the matter is that it is not an easy feat to lose excess weight. When you think about it, how long did it take to get to this point? We're not saying that it is going to be easy, but we will promise you that it will be worth it. Your body will thank you when you are beautiful, and healthy, in and out! Of course, we would never expect you to brave it alone. The follow chapters will be covering some simple mistakes you may be making without realizing that you are jeopardizing yourself!

Hopefully, you have read my first book, "Ketogenic Diet: Quick and Easy Weight Loss Tips with Ketogenic Diet Recipes in 30 Days." In this book, we went into depth on the history of the ketogenic diet is, how your hormones and metabolism works on the diet and all the amazing benefits you can reap from the ketogenic diet. We also went over some of the long and short term effects of the diet. At this point, you should be an expert on the ketogenic and all it offers. Now, you have the information, but something still may be going wrong? Don't worry—this happens to everyone!

In the chapters to follow you will be learning just some of the mistakes you could be making. Dieting is not easy! You are strong and determined. Always remind yourself when you ask yourself why you're putting yourself through this. Remember that you are worth this extra effort. Now, all you need to do is correct some mistakes that you may not even realize you're making. For example, you have most likely been taught most of your life that fat is bad. This is not true! In our ninth chapter, we go over the good and bad of fat! In all honesty, it is something our body needs despite what other diets say. Along with this, we go over some other dieting mistakes you may be making such as miscalculating your calories and calculating your carbohydrates incorrectly.

When these issues were pointed out, to discourage you from dieting. You should realize that everyone makes a mistake at one time or another. It will take a bit of an adjustment to get to your new lifestyle. In fact, we cover this in one of our chapters. Most dieters expect their results in the first week or two. This may not happen for everyone! Our body chemistries are all different. Let's face it; you probably haven't treated your body with as much respect as it deserves up to this point. Now, let's correct those mistakes and get on our way to treating our bodies the right way!

Mistake Number One:
Miscounting Your Calories

The world would be a much easier place to live in if everything was written in black and white. When we diet, we understand that we must measure our calories. But, what is a calorie exactly? Scientifically, a calorie is what measures the amount of energy that is contributed from our food. Our energy is provided by the macronutrients, also known as our carbohydrates, our fats, and proteins that we take in. Did you know that water and micronutrients such as vitamins and minerals do not have calories?

In the modern world, many people turn to relying on calorie-counting tools on their technology to help them out. A few examples of these include "MyFitnessPal," and "LoseIt!" While some of these may seem like they have advantages, they could be leading to your failure. The truth is, there are a lot of misconceptions when it comes to calories and dieting. In fact, while some nutritionists believe that calories in vs. calories out is what matters, other think that it only matters where the calories come from. In the chapter to follow, we will be explaining some misconceptions you may be having with your calorie counting

Calories In vs. Calories Out

It sounds pretty simple, no? Simple is dangerous and incredibly inaccurate. Our body has a complete system. This is exactly why our dieting can't be explained in one sentence! So, what does calorie in mean exactly? It is what we eat! This is very simple. Unlike other organisms, our body cannot metabolize oxygen or sunlight. We get our energy from what we put into our bodies. Now, it is the calories out that gets a bit more confusing. This is because there are several attributes from calories out.

First, we lost calories from our resting energy expenditure. This means that we lose energy simply from our day-to-day physical functions. It takes a lot of energy to live our daily lives and for our bodies to maintain good health. Then, we also lose calories when we digest and process our food. This thermic effect is necessary so we can get the proper nutrients that our body needs to survive. Last, we also burn calories through active energy expenditure. This meaning, calories burned from movement such as walking, jogging, and lifting weights. However, we also burn calories from random activities such as pacing, shivering, and even fidgeting when you're nervous through the day.

Amount and Type of Calorie

It would be very convenient if our calories in and calories out were independent. This way, we could drop our energy intake and maintain the resting metabolic rate. This way, we could burn more energy through digesting food and working out. If this were the case, we would be able to melt the fat right off our body at an excellent and constant rate. If this were the case, we probably wouldn't have such an obesity problem! However, since most of us live in the real world, we must realize that the number of calories we take in and the type of calories consumed will change the energy that we release.

Some of you may be having issues with restricting your calories. What you must realize is when you take calories away, your body will defend itself. It does this by lowering your metabolic rate during spontaneous physical activity. If you wish to counteract this, you will have to reduce your food intake more and move more. The basic concept is to offset the reduced metabolic rate and recreate the movement by consciously fidgeting, twiddling your thumbs, or even tapping your feet. You will have to do this constantly as your body will always try to readjust itself to the issues.

Another factor that people must realize is that whole food will indeed take more energy to process compared to processed foods. In our seventh chapter, we will be going over the importance of eating real food. For example, imagine that there are two sandwiches in front of you. One has whole foods including multigrain bread and cheddar cheese. The other sandwich is made with processed white bread and some package that was labeled "cheese product." Now, imagine that they both have the same number of calories, and mostly the same amount of proteins, fats, and carbohydrates. The group that eats the white bread sandwich will expend about 73 calories as compared to the whole grain group that will expend 137 calories! When you're dieting, that 50% reduction for the thermic effect of your food will make a huge difference! The truth of the matter is, calories in vs. calories out can never be independent of each other.

Less is Not More

When we start a diet, we just think it will be easy as cutting back calories. However, when we consume too few calories, it can backfire and even harm our bodies. When your body has sufficient fuel, it will burn fat even faster. If you take the fuel away, your body loses its ability to function on basic biological processes. This means that your metabolism will slow down so that you can conserve energy. After all, our bodies are wired to survive. Your body needs to adjust so that you don't starve to death. Remember, your body doesn't realize there is a McDonalds around every corner! Even worse, your body will start to break down your muscle tissue for energy rather than fat. When we diet, we want to lose the fat. Instead, if you are taking in too few calories, your body will deteriorate through the muscle mass and bone first.

Understanding calories and metabolism is incredibly important. The threshold where the metabolism slows down is debatable. Some sources have stated that it is at 1200 calories for women and 1800 calories for men but remember that this number will vary thanks to the chemistry of our bodies. While on the ketogenic diet, we suggest cutting around 100 to 200 calories per day if you want to start to lose weight. When you do this, you will safely lose weight and cut calories over a longer period.

Say No to Low-Calorie

Remember that saying not to believe everything you read? This is one of those cases. When a food label says that it is "Low-fat" it only means that you are not eating the real thing. In fact, these foods are probably highly processed and filled with extra sugars, sodium, starch, additives, and other synthetic ingredients you do not need. These are foods that could potentially hinder all of your hard work and effort to lose weight. In fact, some of these processed foods have been known to lead to weight gain! To be safe, avoid anything that says low-calorie or low-fat. As you will be learning in a later chapter, fat is not the enemy! There is a way to lose weight and eat healthy at the same time.

Perfection is Not All That Matters

So, you have counted calorie after calorie you're saying to yourself. But then you step on the scale, and it has gone up. The best advice we can offer you is never to fixate on that number. Your calories in is never going to be accurate. This is for a few different reasons. It is a mistake that everyone makes, you are not alone despite every effort you have done.

First of all, many people tend to underestimate the number of calories they take in depending on the portion size. In fact, in a study done at Cornell, a professor sound that when someone was eating, the more they ate, the less accurate they were. When a person ate a smaller meal, they underestimated their calories by 10%. When a person ate a bigger meal, they underestimated their calories by 40%! Plus, even if you measured your portions correctly, it is impossible to account for the ingredients used in your food.

Finally, it is hard to estimate how our bodies are going to digest and absorb the food we put into our system. This is especially true if the calorie count comes from a nutrition label. Long story short, we are not saying that you should abandon the calorie counting altogether. We suggest keeping track of your food, but the calorie counting isn't as important. Simply maintain the balance of eating well and use calorie counting as a tool of awareness rather than a measurement of your weight loss. This could be step one to losing weight the way you want!

Mistake Number Two: Measuring Your Ketones

As you probably realize, ketones are super beneficial to helping the fat metabolize in our body. When we restrict the amount of carbohydrate we put into our body, this is how we lower the blood sugar and insulin levels in our body. When the insulin levels begin to fall, our body still needs energy. At this point, a fatty acid flows from the nasty fat cells and into our bloodstream so we can begin to metabolize. As you will recall, this process is known as beta-oxidation. At the end of this process, we are left with a molecule known as acetyl-CoA. As more of the fatty acids are metabolized, the amount of these acetyl-CoA rises. Through this process, a metabolic feedback loop begins, and our liver shells stop any excess acetyl-CoA into ketogenesis, also known as the reason our body makes ketone bodies.

Remember that when these ketone bodies are created, the liver dumps them into our blood stream and then they are taken to our heart and skeletal muscles. On top of this, our brain begins to use these ketones as fuel when the levels are high enough to cross that barrier. As you will recall, there are three major types of the ketone bodies that have been presented in our blood stream. These are the Acetoacetate, the B-hydroxybutyrate, and the acetone. This is why it is imperative to begin your low carbohydrate intake. When you do, your insulin levels will lower, and your ketone bodies will start up to 50% of the energy your body needs to function. When carbohydrates are restricted, your body stops relying on glucose and can use ketogenesis to burn fuel for your cells.

So, where could you be going wrong with measuring your ketones? It could be a few different things. One, you could not be measuring at all and just expecting your body to do the work for you. As you will be learning, this could be harmful to your health. Two, you could be measuring the wrong way or you not understand the concept of ketosis and how to stay in it. Don't worry; we will help you along the way. Last, if you measure your ketone bodies, it may be time to change up your method. We will be offering you four different alternatives to make sure you get on the right track!

Ketoacidosis

Despite what some professionals have said, it is now believed that nutritional ketosis is not the same as ketoacidosis. You may be asking yourself, what is ketoacidosis? It doesn't sound exquisite! The truth of the matter is, it is just as bad as it sounds. This ketoacidosis is a very dangerous condition that has been associated with having a lack of insulin in your body. Some people that have been known to experience this state are diabetics who don't make enough insulin. This illness causes the blood sugar to rise about 200 mg/dL and can be very dangerous.

What you must realize is that this feeling is not nutritional ketosis. If this happens, your ketone bodies could rise above 10-25mM. Remember that nutritional ketosis ranges between 0.5-3.0mM. But, why does this happen? It could be because there is no insulin to stop fat burning. When this happens, the fatty acids flow out of your cells and converted into the ketone bodies and placed into your blood stream. When there are higher levels of ketone bodies in the bloodstream, it becomes too acidic and can create health issues including fruiter breath, hyperventilation, low blood pressure, dehydration, and vomiting. If left untreated, this could lead to a coma or death through either respiratory failure, brain swelling or even other tissue damage. This is why learning to measure ketones correctly is incredibly important.

Best Ways to Measure Ketones

1. Blood Ketone MeterSome believe that this is the most accurate way to measure the ketone bodies, especially BHB. The meter can determine the level of ketones in your blood. It should be noted that this gadget is a bit pricey. In retrospect, the meter can cost about $40 alone with the strips costing about $5 a piece. If you wish to test yourself on a daily basis, this could cost about $150 plus the extra $40 for the meter. On the one hand, it is nice to have an accurate measurement, on the other, you could be using that extra money on food for your diet. If the number is vital to you, the blood ketone meter is most likely your best option.

2. Urine Ketone Strips

3. These are also known as Ketostix or Uriscan. We wish to make it understood that these are not always extremely accurate. In fact, they may not work for some people. These strips are only able to show you the excess ketone bodies that you have excreted through your urine. This counts the number of acetoacetates. However, it does not tell you anything about the BHB in your bloodstream. In most cases, they are probably higher than the level the strip shows you. It should also be noted that these strips do not measure all of the types of ketones that your body produces. They only measure the acetoacetate, and this will change

depending on how long you have been in ketosis. This number will change especially when you become keto-adapted. At this point, you will begin to excrete fewer ketone bodies in your urine compared to before. This could mean that you have a high number of ketones in your body and none in your urine. You can see where this could become dangerous. This level will also change depending on how hydrated you are. If you take a lot of water in, it could dilute the concentration of ketones in your urine. While it is important to stay hydrated, it could affect the reading of your urine strip.

4. Some people have used the urine ketone strips to test if they are sensitive to certain foods that claim to be keto-friendly. They do this to see if it is due to a particular food that is having an adverse effect on their weight loss. The positive of these tests is that they are both cheap and easy to use. In most stores, the strips are $10 for 50 strips. This means that it costs about $6 a month so you can test yourself daily. If these do not work for you, do not be discouraged. There are three other ways to measure your ketone bodies accurately.

5. Breathalyzer If you are looking for a cheap and non-invasive way to measure your ketone bodies, the breathalyzer may be the best option for you. Remember that Acetone is a ketone body that results from the acetoacetate when it is broken down. The breath test will measure the acetone concentration on your breath. This is an easy and cheap way to test your ketones. However, it should be noted that the number of ketones on your breath may not always correlate with the ketones in your body. This number can be affected by factors such as alcohol consumption and drinking water.

6. Observation: If you don't want to take any of these fancy tests from above or simply just can't afford it, you could always listen to your bodies signals to find out if you're in ketosis or not. When you are in ketosis, some dieters have claimed to smell of acetone. You may be asking yourself, what is the smell of acetone? Most of the time, it is sensed in the breath, urine, or even your sweat. Some people refer to this stage of smelling "fruity." If you sense any of these signs, you are probably in ketosis. However, to stay on the safe side, we suggest measuring with one of the tests from above.

Staying in Ketosis

For some people, staying in ketosis is the hardest part of the diet. In fact, if you consume more than 100 grams of protein and more than 60 grams of carbohydrates during most of your diet, it will be a guaranteed stop on your process to nutritional ketosis. At this point, your brain will not be able to use the ketone bodies in your bloodstream efficiently. Why does this happen, though? Studies have found that 56% of excess protein is metabolized into glucose. This will have a huge impact on your ketosis. If you want to stay in ketosis, there are a few different tricks you can try to get you on your way.

1. Eat less protein

2. Eat more healthy fat

3. Cut out the carbohydrates

4. Measure in an accurate way

5. Try a fat fast if you've been on a diet a while

6. Learn how to relax

7. Give time to adapt to the diet

8. Check your portions

Mistake Number Three:
Scale Obsession Issues

Most people have a sick obsession with their scale. That tiny number in front of you determines so much for you and can either make or break your day. As you read this, you are probably thinking of all the times you've been motivated or discouraged due to your scale. The real question is, how many times do you weigh yourself? Do you measure on a daily basis? Or perhaps you even weight yourself more than once a day. While of course, it is great to measure yourself from time to time to make sure you are on the right track, it is time to stop obsessing over the number! The number on the scale does not reflect your fitness level, your progress, or your inner beauty. There are ways to create a healthy relationship with your scale and believe us; it is necessary.

Setting an Increment

As we mentioned earlier, it is not healthy to weigh yourself every single day. This is something that will hinge your weight loss when you are stressing over it on a daily basis. It is important that you find the simple balance of weighing yourself. You need to monitor whether you are on the upward or downward of your weight goal. When you set a particular time increment, it will prevent you from obsessing over the numbers every day. Instead, choose to measure yourself once a week or so. Remember that the number on the scale will change depending on your diet and your daily activity. We learned this is especially now that we realize that calorie in doesn't always equal calorie out!

Be Realistic

You are on a diet. You should be very proud of your efforts thus far. However, there are many people out there who get a number stuck in their head and then obsess over this number until they reach their goal. Perhaps it is a number that they saw on someone else or a number they were a long time ago. When you set your weight goal, try to be realistic about your number. Some weights may not be healthy for your body type. Also, remember that this number will change as you develop muscle. Muscle does weight more than fat. When you choose your number, account for the amount of muscle you will have. Perhaps try adding 5 pounds to your number.

Weight Fluctuates

If you are one of those people who measure themselves every day, you may notice that the number moves A LOT. This is because many factors can affect your weight. If you are a lady, your cycle can change your weight. Your weight will also vary depending on if you've had a lot of salts, if you just ate recently, and even the last time you had a bowel movement! Gross, but true. This is just another reason we discourage daily weight measurement. There's no need to freak out if you're a few pounds heavier than you were the day before.

At the end of the day, the basic concept is not to obsess over the number. As long as you are following the diet, eating correctly, and keeping yourself in check, you are on the right path. There are some ways to develop a healthy relationship with your scale, so dieting isn't so miserable for you.

Tip Number One: Eat Good, Feel Good

Remember that eating well is the central concept of the ketogenic diet. While exercise may be substantial, healthy eating will dictate how you feel through the day and will eventually show on your scale. Essentially, you do not want to eat processed foods. Remember that they are filled with sodium, sugar, and saturated fat that will just make you feel sluggish. Stop making these poor decisions. Bad decisions will only lead to other bad decisions. Instead, try to focus on eating nutrient foods like lean proteins, fruits, and vegetables. Try your best to treat your body the way it deserves to be treated. For a safe rule, fuel your body with foods that contain the least number of ingredients. Choose fresh whenever possible to gain the most from your diet.

Tip Number Two: Focus On Feeling

For lack of better words, screw what the scale says! Have you been eating well, resting well, and working out on a regular basis? If you feel great, don't let a number on a scale tell you otherwise. Don't sweat it! Remember that your scale could be off for a few reasons. Whether your weight is fluctuating, perhaps you've gained muscle, or maybe it's the scale itself! That number is not a label you need to slap on yourself. If you've been working hard the way you should be, you will be losing weight. It may take longer than you would like but remember to stick to the plan. This new, healthy lifestyle will be worth it when you reach your goal. Don't allow your goal to be a certain number on the scale. You will never reach it if that is the case!

Tip Number Three: Be Confident

When you feel good, you look good! You are given one body to live in, feel confident in your skin. When you believe in yourself, others will too. When you are confident, you may find that you become empowered in other parts of your life whether it be at home or work. Try to engage in an activity that sparks your imagination. Put on clothes that make you feel great. By making just a few changes, you may find your whole attitude changing. Remember that you do not need a scale to tell you otherwise. While it is ok to measure every once in a while, the number on your scale should not take over your whole life.

Other Ways to Measure Weight

If the scale stresses you out too much, don't worry. Luckily for you, there are plenty of other ways to gauge the success of your weight loss. Remember that if you are working hard, the weight is going to come off. Just make sure you're doing all the right things and give it time. Here are just a few other ways to measure your weight loss:

1. Progress Photos

2. Ideally, you should wear the same outside and stand in the same place and the same way. While some people do this once a month, feel free to do it whenever you feel comfortable. This way, you can notice small changes you may not notice if you look at yourself every day. Also, ditch the "before and after" lingo. A healthy lifestyle is a lifelong process. Remember always to improve, and you will keep that annoying weight off!

3. Track Your Habits

   The number on the scale isn't going to be the only thing that will change. We want you to keep a journal of aspects you are adding to your life. For example, track when you eat that healthy meal or go for the walk you've been thinking about. When you track your new healthy habits, you will be able to track your consistency as well.

4. Put on the Pants

5. For some of us, we start dieting when our clothes start getting a little tight. We suggest your clothes on and seeing how they feel. When the pants fit, this is a good sign that you are losing weight. Even better, try putting on pants that may be a few years old. If your clothes are more comfortable, this is much greater than the number going down on the scale. This will be a sure sign that you are losing fat versus the scale that can change depending on the fluid shifts in your body.

6. Talk It Out

7. When you change your lifestyle, it doesn't need to be alone. Choose a friend to go along the journey with. Perhaps choose a monthly or weekly time to give each other positive feedback. Remember to choose a friend that is going to be positive but also honest. It is important that your comments are always constructive. You must keep an open mind if you want to make a change. Remember that you are going to make mistakes, that's why you're here isn't it? Your friend will be able to call you out if they think you could change

something to benefit your diet and weight loss. I'm sure they would expect the same from you!

8. Other Numbers

9. Yes, there are other numbers aside from just the numbers on the scale. We are talking about your fat percentage measurement. Remember that it is entirely possible to reduce your body fat and still weigh the same. This stands especially true if you are gaining lean muscle! When you measure your bodies such as the waist, hips, and upper thighs, this will give you a number to track that may be a bit more accurate compared to the scale. Either way, just make sure you have a reasonable way to track your weight loss to make sure you're in the right direction of going down!

Mistake Number Four:
Fear or Fat

You've been counting your calories, eating healthy, and keeping your body in ketosis by following all the rules. You either aren't losing weight or your gaining it. What gives? The truth is, it could be your thoughts that are throwing you off the weight loss wagon! Did you know that the fear of regaining weight is incredibly common? In fact, many people are less than optimistic when they start dieting again. This attitude is what needs to change if you are going to lose weight. Often, diets are associated with negative attitudes. If you want to lose weight, you need to get over that fear of fat!

Causes of Pocrescophobia

This question can be a bit tricky. This is because the issue will vary depending on the individual. While this is most commonly a symptom of Bulimia or Anorexia, there are other reasons this phobia can be created. When you obsess over gaining weight, you are most likely going to gain weight. Trauma is one reason that a person could develop a fear of getting fat. This could be due to the fact the individual gained weight in the past or experienced someone else gains weight. Unfortunately, obesity causes some health problems including death. If someone lost a loved one due to weight loss, this could create the fear of gaining weight themselves.

One could also develop a fear of getting fat if they have a low self-esteem. This stands especially true in our society that values beauty in the thin. If you are someone who buys into these messages, it is no wonder you have a fear of gaining weight. Nobody in their right mind wants to be deemed undesirable by their peers. If you think you suffer from any of these causes, see if your fears match the symptoms. We do not want you to worry. You are not too far gone. We do not want your fears to hinder your weight loss. We promise that when you look at the big picture, your lifestyle changes on the ketogenic diet will make all of the difference.

Symptoms of Pocrescophobia

This issue is so common; it even has a name! The irrational fear of gaining weight is known as Pocrescophobia. Most of the time, this fear comes from people who feel pressure to fit in with others. Most commonly, it is seen within dancers, aesthetic athletes, and especially woman. It should be noted that men have been known to have this phobia as well. How can you tell if you have this fear or not? It can be hard to say as the symptoms will change depending on the person. It can vary due to several factors including personality, the level of fear, and state of mind. You may have this phobia if you obsess over weight loss, obsess over the scale, avoid food, or even feel guilty when you eat food.

Unfortunately, this fear of food has led to other eating disorders. These include anorexia and bulimia. If you weren't already away, Anorexia is when a person does not eat. On the other hand, bulimia occurs when a person overeats and then forces themselves to purge afterward. These diseases have also been linked with people who exercise in excess. For those who have this phobia, they may panic if they gain a little weight. Panic attacks include breathing difficulties, fainting, dizziness, tingling, sweating, feeling of loss of control, chest pain, or a rapid heart rate. Some may be asking, what causes this phobia in the first place?

Treatment for Pocrescophobia

If you want to get over your fear of gaining weight, it is important that you realize the science behind gaining weight. Luckily, it is quite simple. If you want to lose weight, you must eat less. You have to burn more calories than you take in. By following the ketogenic diet and eating the correct foods, you will be able to lose weight. Remember that this diet was formed to help boost your metabolism. When your body is functioning the way it is meant to, running off ketone bodies, you will lose weight like you desire. Your metabolism plays a huge factor in the way your body uses calories. By understanding the science, it may help you get over this irrational fear.

It should be noted that the treatment of this fear will vary depending on the individual. For most, therapy is a great start. Several forms can be used to understand and treat the fear. We suggest a type of social therapy to help individuals build their self-esteem along the way. Remember a major part of looking great is feeling great!

If therapy isn't in your cards, there is always medication that can be used to help the anxiety. Medicine also takes care of the symptoms of panic attacks if you are easily subjected to these issues. If medication isn't your cup of tea, there are rehab centers that are specifically for those who have an eating disorder. This way, you have a supportive environment to express your feelings and be able to share your fears with those who suffer from the same condition. Either way, realize that you are never alone. Having food-related fears is incredibly common. What is important is that you recognize these issues and try to fix them so you can move on to a better, healthier lifestyle.

Mistake Number Five:
Protein: Good and Bad

As you probably know, protein is a huge portion of the Ketogenic diet. However, remember that everything can be good in moderation. Some of you may be taking in too much protein for your own good! According to The National Institute of Medicine Food and Nutrition Board, adults should only be consuming about 0.8 grams of protein per kilogram of their body weight. This is about 8 grams of protein per 20 pounds of body weight. While protein is excellent for helping people lose weight, remember that your health should always come first! Below, we will be going over some of the signs that you may be eating too much protein. If this is the case, you will want to consider making some changes to your diet to help you lose weight in a healthy manner.

Sign Number One: Gaining Weight for 'No Reason.'

When you are on the Ketogenic diet, you should be keeping track of your consumption in some form. When you go back through your days, check to see if you have been sticking to your diet. If you haven't been indulging in sweets and snacks yet your weight seems to be creeping up; it is probably the protein. When you eat more protein than your diet needs, this protein will begin to add excess calories. Therefore, over time, you will start to gain weight which is exactly the opposite of what you want! If you seem to be gaining weight, try cutting the protein back for a few days and see if the weight drops.

Sign Number Two: Rising Cholesterol Levels

Research has shown that the amount of protein you eat has a direct correlation to your cholesterol levels. This is because high-protein foods contain a lot more cholesterol than you probably expect. This is an unwanted condition, especially because it can lead to other medical problems including both stroke and heart attack. Overall, you should not be getting any more than 200 milligrams of cholesterol per day. Be sure to watch how much protein you are consuming so you can remain healthy and can lose weight.

Sign Number Three: Dehydrated All The Time

When you bulk up on protein, this is what helps create the ketones in our body. Through this process of excreting the ketones, there is a lot of water loss through the kidneys. When this happens, your body will become dehydrated. When you have too much protein, it correlates to dehydration. Now that you are aware of this process, you can start to drink more water so you can keep the flow of ketones running through your body in a healthy manner.

Sign Number Four: Osteoporosis

When we take in a lot of protein, our body begins to excrete more calcium in our kidneys. When this happens, it increases the risk for osteoporosis. If you weren't aware, this is a condition that causes your bones to become weak. If you have been feeling in pain since you have started the diet, you may want to get checked out by a professional. We want to remind you that your health must always come first. True, losing weight can help you get to that point, but not every diet is for every person. Please stop immediately if you are suffering in any way, shape or form.

Other Troubles from Too Much Protein

If you take in too much protein, it could lead to some other serious health issues. First, you could develop a kidney disease. When you take in too much protein, that means you are taking in more nitrogen as well. When this happens, it will place more strain on the kidneys than necessary. As a reaction, your body expels this nitrogen in your urine. If you already have kidney disease, the Ketogenic diet is most likely not for you.

High protein diets have been known to cause kidney stones as well. As we mentioned earlier, the more protein you take in, the more calcium is excreted through the kidneys. When this happens, it increases the risk of osteoporosis. In other cases, too much protein was also linked to an increased cancer risk. This is why it is important not to eat too much protein. If you follow the diet correctly, you will only reap the rewards of the diet and avoid these serious possibilities.

Benefits of Eating Protein

As you know, eating protein is crucial for your weight loss. However, other amazing benefits eating protein will bring into your life. Have you always struggled with having a slow metabolism and have issues losing weight? You may be eating too little protein! A lack of protein has also been related to other symptoms including having issues building any muscle, having very low energy levels, having issues with mood swings, having a low immunity, and even suffering from muscle, bone, and joint pain. If you have any of the symptoms from above, the Ketogenic diet will do wonders for your life.

One of the benefits you will get from eating protein is helping improve your muscle mass. When you eat enough, your body will begin to build and primary muscles which in return will support your ligaments, tendon, and other body tissue. This is especially important if you are active. When we train, we are tearing and damaging our muscle tissue. When you eat enough protein, it helps the body repair and grows back even stronger.

Protein in the diet will also manage your weight. How? It fills you up! When you eat protein, it will help you feel fuller, quicker, and in return will stop you from overeating. Overall, studies have found that it is exceptionally easy to eat carbohydrates. This is even more so true if these carbs are sweetened and refined. At the same time, the protein will also help prevent any muscle loss as we had already mentioned.

While the benefits of protein could go on and on, we want to mention that eating protein can help improve your mood1 this is because the amino acids found in protein naturally balance your hormones. In fact, it acts as a natural remedy if you suffer from anxiety. If you ask me, all of these are fantastic reasons to take in more protein in your diet. Just remember that moderation is what matters.

Best Sources of Protein

While there is a downside of protein when eaten in excess, protein is still vital for your diet and weight loss. Below, we will give you a list of high protein foods to help you on the road to success:

- **Fish**

- Try to stick with wild fish such as catfish, cod, and flounder. Other great choices include salmon, trout, and even tuna!

- **Eggs**

- If you can, try to get your eggs free-range. The best part is that you can prepare eggs in various ways. This keeps your diet different and delicious.

- **Meat**

- When possibly, get animal products that are grass fed. This will make sure that your meal has a better fatty acid. Stick with animals including Goat, lamb, veal, beef, and other wild game.

- **Poultry**

- This is another food product that should be either organic or free-range. These include duck, chicken, quail, and even pheasant. All these are delicious choices to cook up for lunch or dinner.

- **Pork**

- When you are choosing your meat, watch for any additives. If possible, try to get this as fresh as possible. Stick with anything from ham to pork chops.

Mistake Number Six: Carbohydrate Calculations

If you are on the Ketogenic diet, you are most likely already aware that carbohydrates are not good for your system. This is why they are such a small percentage of your macronutrients. But, what is a carbohydrate exactly? Normally, it is a nutrient that is used by your body. This nutrient contains 4 kilocalories of energy. When your body converts this carbohydrate, it turns it into glucose to keep you running. What you may not know is that the conversion can either happen slow or quick depending on the type of food. The rate at which the conversion occurs is the Glycemic Index.

While this may sound a bit complicated, it is pretty simple to explain. All you need to know is that a slower conversion is better for your system. When faster food is converted, your blood sugar levels will rise quicker. Apparently, wrong. When this happens, insulin rushes into your bloodstream and stops fat loss altogether. If you can gain control of this insulin secretion (like the Ketogenic diet does), it helps mobilize the fat from your fat cells. When this happens, you will drop weight.

Non-Impact Carbohydrate

Simply, a non-impact carb has a small effect on your blood sugar level. These are the carbs that will be allowed on your diet. Mostly, these low-carb foods are made of fiber. Fiber is indigestible and passes through your system easily. Mostly, these are found in vegetables, whole grains, and fruits.

Effective Carbohydrates

As you could guess, these carbohydrates do have effect on your blood sugar levels. This is precisely why effective carbohydrates are limited in your diet. This will help keep your blood sugar and insulin levels under control. The effective carbohydrates are broken down into simple and complex carbs. The simple carbohydrates are rapidly converted while the complex carbohydrates take longer to convert into glucose. Just remember that these should be limited altogether if you wish to lose weight.

Net Carbohydrates vs. Total Carbohydrates

In simple terms, net carbs are your total carbs without the fiber. Remember that fiber comes in two different types, soluble and insoluble. Most people on the Ketogenic diet use their net carbs because they view dietary fiber as ineffective in the system. Therefore, your body doesn't derive calories from it. While it is noted that some dieters believe this, the claim isn't 100% accurate. It appears only insoluble fiber cannot be absorbed. Try to count your net carbohydrates if you want your calculations to be accurate.

Signs You Are Eating Too Many Carbohydrates

Now that you understand the carbohydrate basics, could they be holding you back from weight loss? Studies have debated if carbs are even needed for human nutrition. Unfortunately, carbohydrates are delicious. However, they can have an adverse impact on several different aspects including weight, digestion, immunity, and even energy. Below, we will be listing some of the signs you could be experiencing if you are eating way too many carbohydrates.

1. Your weight is fluctuating more quickly than normal

2. You have crazy energy fluctuations throughout the day

3. You feel irritable and light-headed when you are hungry

4. You are craving sweet treats all of the time

5. You are craving starchy foods for no reason

6. You have a hard time controlling sugar and carbohydrates in your diet

7. You turn to sugar and carbohydrates when you are feeling depressed or tired

8. You feel exhausted after eating a carb-heavy meal

9. You gain weight despite eating "healthy" carbohydrates

10. You feel foggy after eating

Low-Carb Flu

If you are following the ketogenic diet as you should be, you have probably heard of the dreaded low-carb flu. This happens when you dramatically reduce your carb intake. This transition period can be a bit rough, but it will be worth it. Some of the symptoms of the low-carb flu include: feeling fuzzy, suffering from throbbing headaches, feeling exhausted and irritable for no reason, feeling hungry all of the time, craving everything but mostly carbohydrates.

You may be thinking to yourself, but this diet is supposed to be making me feel better! Do not worry. Not everyone experiences the low-carb flu. It is a short-term pain for a long-term gain, remember that! Luckily for you, there are several ways to blast right through the horrible flu and get your body into a state of ketosis.

First, you will want to eat more fat. While this sounds like it will counteract your weight loss, remember that you are trying to replace your carbohydrates with fat as your primary source of energy. The goal is to get at least 60% of your calories from this fat. Later in the book, we will be going over the good and bad of fat and what you should be eating. Another way to help get over the low-flu carb is to make sure you're not eating too much protein. This is something we already covered.

Another fantastic way to get over the flu is to avoid any foods that have sweeteners or sugar-free in the title. While there are claims that they are safe for the low-carb diet, they should be avoided when you first get into your low carb diet. You want to break away from your addiction to sugar. If you are consuming treats that taste sweet, you are just going to confuse your system. More than likely, you will just trigger your body and create stronger cravings. You will want to avoid this as you want to move forward, not back.

Gaining a Healthy Relationship with Carbohydrates

It can be next to impossible to cut carbohydrates out from your diet. Why should you? Everything is fine in moderation, remember that? Instead, reach for the foods that are green leafy vegetables and have healthy fats. When you do this, these foods fill you with nutrients. This way, you won't go looking for unhealthy foods when your body is happy and healthy. You may be asking yourself, well what about cheat days? Some people wonder if they can actually benefit for faster weight loss. While some claim that this could help overcome any weight loss plateaus, it will vary depending on the individual. If you do include a cheat day while on the ketogenic diet, you may feel you put weight on due to the water retention. When you go back to your low-carb diet, you will probably feel the effect immediately. While carb-days could work for some days, we highly recommend against it. Instead, try to include some more weight training if your weight loss has stopped.

Another great way to help your body tolerate more carbohydrates is by exercising. When you move, at least you will be burning any calories you did take in. There is nothing that effects weight loss more than sitting around and eating foods that you shouldn't be. No matter what your relationship may be with carbohydrates, be sure to give yourself a fresh start. Find the right carbohydrate level for yourself and check your ketogenic guide to help you on your way to becoming a happier and healthier you!

Mistake Number Seven:
Issues with Fake Food

You may be asking, what do you mean by fake food? The word "processed" generally causes some confusion. This is meaning that most foods that are consumed are handled in some way. However, there is a difference between mechanical processing such as cutting apples from the tree or churning milk into butter and a chemical processing. Food that has been chemically processed with other ingredients and artificial substances are horrible for you. Here are just some of the ways that fake food is terrible for your health:

1. Fake Food and Over Consumption

   It is part of our nature to want to eat food. Thanks to evolution, we have taste buds that help us navigate through the natural environment. Naturally, our appetite will go for foods that are either fatty, sweet, or salty. In earlier times, we needed these nutrients for energy so that we could survive. Now, it isn't as necessary. While processed foods may be rewarding to our brains, it isn't as rewarding to our hips. Remember that when you are grocery shopping next time!

2. High Fructose Corn Syrup and Sugar

   As you could have probably guessed, processed foods are loaded with excess sugar and high fructose corn syrup. These empty calories can cause some serious damage to your inside and forget about having a metabolism. When you take in too much sugar, it leads to issues such as insulin resistance and increased levels of cholesterol. On top of that, high sugar consumption is associated with obesity, diabetes, and other heart diseases. This is just another reason to avoid the fake food!

3. Artificial Ingredients

Let's be honest, does that even sound healthy? Most of the time when you are looking at packaged food, you can't read half of the 'ingredients' used. This is because they aren't found in actual food! Most processed foods contain preservatives, colorants, flavors, and textures. While these chemicals have been tested for safety, the stamp of approval should be taken with a grain of salt. Why put the fake in when you can get healthy, real food in your system?

4. No Nutrients

Compared to unprocessed foods, the fake foods offer little to no nutrients that your body needs. Most of the time, companies will add synthetic minerals and vitamins to the food due to the fact they were lost during processing! These are not a good replacement from the nutrients you could be getting from real food. You need these nutrients to keep your body in a healthy manner.

5. Fake Food Addiction As we mentioned earlier, fake food is very rewarding for your brain. Did you know that people can get addicted to junk food? It is believed that this is a huge issue in today's society, where people simply cannot stop eating these disgusting foods no matter how hard they try! In some studies, sugar and junk food activate the same brain areas as cocaine does.

While it may not be at the same danger level, it could be preventing you from losing weight as you would like!

Benefits of Eating Real Food

Luckily, getting over your fake food addiction is a quick fix. All you need to do is eat real food! Yes, it is as simple as that. When you switch to a real food diet, you will begin to notice the health improvements in an instant. While of course being on the Ketogenic diet can be challenging, it will be worth it. Plus, there are amazing health benefits that occur aside from just the weight loss.

When you begin to eat unprocessed foods, you may find that your mood will become more stabilized. This could be because you have more energy! Now that your body isn't running on glucose from carbohydrates, you will feel more energized through the day and not suffer from those energy crashes! You may also find that your brain will begin to clear. If you have been forgetful lately, it may be the fake food! When you eat real foods, that cloud above your head will probably lift so you can function better through the day.

Eating unprocessed foods will also lead to stronger nails, healthier hair, and less bloat in your tummy! When you eat more nutrient dense foods, it will help you keep the weight off and become more regular during your bathroom trips. Say goodbye if you suffer from constipation and hello to a healthier schedule. When you eat better, you will feel better!

Mistake Number Eight:
Fat is Not the Enemy

If you need a mantra on your diet, let it be "Fat is not the enemy." Unfortunately, fat gets an atrocious rep. This is also the reason most strive to eliminate the fat from their diets altogether. The truth is, you are just eating the wrong type of fat. Yes. Bad fat can lead to all sorts of health issues including heart disease, diabetes, stroke, and high cholesterol. At all costs, you want to avoid saturated and trans fats. What you do need in your system is monounsaturated fats and polyunsaturated fats. These two are excellent when eaten in moderation. Most of your ketogenic diet will be made of these fats for such reasons.

Another important nutrition to get into your diet is essential fatty acids such as omega-3. These help your body out in ways from fighting dementia and even reducing inflammation. You will want to cut back on foods that are rich in omega-6 as most American's have an unhealthy amount in their diet. It is all about finding that perfect balance to keep yourself healthy. So, how do you know if you aren't getting enough fat in your diet? There are a few signs you can look for!

1. Anger and Depression

    You may not know, but omega-3 acids are very effective to prevent and manage depression. If you have crazy mood swings, you may have to up your omega-3 intake. You can find these in fatty fish, chia seeds, and even flax seeds. You may find that they make a huge difference. In one study done, those who took cod liver oil were 30% less likely to suffer from symptoms of depression.

2. Dry Skin

3. Is your skin dry and itchy? Reach for the olive oil and avocados. You may need to give your body fatty acids to help produce oil in your glands. This is your bodies way of naturally moisturizing itself. When you maintain healthy skin membranes, your body will produce lipids. Lipids are the skin barriers that stop water from escaping through your pores. When you have enough, it keeps your skin hydrated and beautiful.

4. Always Hungry

You may think this is from your diet, but it could be your body's need for fat! Research has shown that dietary fat helps you feel full and in return can regulate your appetite. Try your best to up your polyunsaturated fatty acids to keep yourself full and healthy. While this isn't a free card to eat as much fat as you would like, remember that a little can go a long way, especially when it comes to fats.

5. Lack of Energy

Most people begin to feel tired at some point in the afternoon. If you are one that crashes in the middle of the day, you may need to up your fat intake. Out of the three macronutrients (carbohydrates, fats, and proteins), it is the fat that has the most concentrated source of energy. When eaten with other foods, fat slows digestion down and improves your insulin sensitivity. When this happens, there is less of a chance you will suffer from a sugar crash.

6. Foggy Mind

If you have issues concentrating or remembering, you will need more omega-4 fatty acids. They are crucial for both your mental and your memory performance. When you have these fats, it helps build cell membranes in your brain and enables the fibers in your brain to carry messages faster. This is another reason it is important to balance your omega-3 and omega-6 fatty acids.

How to Eat More Good Fat

There is no reason that low-carb eating can't be delicious! When you eat the right fat, it can be filling, healthy, and delicious. While it can be a challenge to people who don't like the idea of putting fat in their diet, here are just some ways you can incorporate fat into your diet to help you lose weight and become healthy.

Cook with Fat

Fat can change the flavor of your dish altogether. Luckily, this can add variety to your meals so that you never get bored! Whether you drizzle them over your vegetables or sauté them in your favorite fat, we always suggest experimenting with new favorite combinations. Some fats you should be cooking with include: butter, coconut oil, olive oil, peanut oil, avocado oil, nut oils, sesame oil, and even lard.

Go Full Fat

As we have mentioned repeatedly, avoid the foods that are labeled low-fat and fat-free. There is no reason to go nonfat when they can benefit your weight loss journey. When you are grocery shopping, think about filling your fridge with whole foods. Try to incorporate delicious foods like eggs and avocados. Another great alternative is fatty cuts of meat. These are delicious and contain healthy fats that will be fantastic for any meal.

Garnish Your Meals

Your whole meal doesn't need to be one big plate of fat. Sometimes it's nice just to top your meals with fat to add some nutrients and flavor. Try shredded parmesan, smoked Gouda cheese, crumbled feta cheese, avocado, bacon, ground sausage, pine nuts, stuffed green olives, flaked coconut and more. Whether you are adding them to salads or your meal just needs some extra spice, you can add these to any dish!

Mistake Number Nine:
Exercising On A Ketogenic Diet

Most diets claim that if you want to lose weight, you need to eat less and exercise more. To most people, this means running on the treadmill until they are about to drop. However, when most people do this, they will quickly become exhausted and will not lose weight the way they would like. This is because they are putting more stress on their body. Studies have shown that there is an accelerated aging process of the cells when there is excess stress placed on the body. If you increase exercise and decrease calories, you will be doing more harm than good to your body.

Most people are on the keto diet because when you can naturally eat less when your appetite is suppressed. So, is exercise necessary to lose weight? If you are just looking to lose weight, the keto diet is all you need. However, there are some benefits to doing some moderate exercise. Some of these health benefits include:

1. Improved Immunity

2. Improved Bone Mineral Density

3. Improved Insulin Sensitivity

4. Anti-aging Benefits

5. Brain Health

6. Cardiovascular Health

Ditch the Cardio

If you would like to exercise, we suggest low-intensity cardio. These activities include hiking, walking, swimming, or even cycling. The issue with society is that people use cardio as their only fat-burning tool. The fact of the matter is, you cannot use prolonged cardio if you want to lose fat. Firstly, it could lead to chronic cardio. When this happens, it will make you hungrier. When you are hungrier, you are more likely to eat more. You will want to avoid increasing your appetite, especially if you want to lose weight.

Chronic cardio has also been known to raise a stress hormone called cortisol. This hormone is in charge of storing fat in your stomach area. In the long run, excess cardio could lead to leptin resistance which is why your body has an appetite and weight regulation. When the leptin begins to resist, your appetite will increase, and your weight loss journey will be doomed.

Instead, you will want to try some weight training or high-intensity interval training. While the number of how long you should exercise varies, some say that you should do moderate exercise for twenty minutes, three or more days a week. Now you may be saying to yourself, "Won't lifting weights make me bulky?" If you are a woman, no. Women just do not have the same hormones as men do. Yes, you will become more defined, but you will not become masculine.

If lifting weights aren't your cup of tea, high-intensity interval training may be an excellent choice for you. This technique uses alternate bursts of anaerobic exercises to give you a full body workout. In fact, you can burn more calories in less time compared to a prolonged cardio session. Long story short, exercising is suggested but just like your diet, everything should be done in moderation. You do not need to exercise every day to lose weight. You will want to make sure that you give your body enough rest days to recover and allow yourself to get enough sleep.

Most people underestimate how important sleep is for weight loss. When you are sleep deprived, you are more likely to get late night munchies and your hunger hormones that normally regulate your appetite will get all out of whack. Make sure you avoid the food temptations by getting enough sleep in your schedule. Remember that it is important to eat right, sleep right, and exercise. At the end of the day, your body will thank you for taking such good care of it.

Mistake Number Ten: Allowing Adaption Time

Yes, getting used to a new lifestyle can be tough. If you are starting out on the Ketogenic diet, you may have heard about keto-adaption. While it may sound a bit intimidating, we are here to teach you about what it is and how to overcome it. Yes, it may be a bit of a struggle, but just think of all the benefits you will get from this diet. It will be worth it.

So, what is keto-adaption? It is the process of shifting your slow metabolism from relying on glucose, to relying on fat sources for its fuel. This is beneficial because the fat will increase oxidation and will help your body to produce the ketones that we keep mentioning. Remember that ketones are a significant source of fuel for your body. As these ketones can be used in both the tissue and the brain, it also makes it so beneficial for your body.

During Keto-adaption

There are two different stages of the keto-adaption. Within the first few days of your new diet, your body will still be running on the glucose it has stored. In all honesty, this will probably be the toughest part of the process. After years of consuming fake foods and sugar, you need to break the cycle of metabolizing through glucose. In the first few days, the ketone production isn't significant enough to turn to fat metabolism. However, you may experience water loss in the first few days. As you lose the water weight, the keto diet will lower the insulin levels and allows the excess fluid to be released. You may notice weight loss, but it should be noted that this is most likely just water loss, you haven't lost any fat, yet.

Once the glycogen has run out, this is when you will begin to produce the ketones. This is when it will be easy to measure the ketones. If you need a reminder, please visit the chapter from earlier to go over how to measure your ketones in the most accurate manner. It will be at this point that ketones are available to use as fuel. As you produce more ketones, the more your body and your brain will rely on them for energy. At this point, your body will begin to depend on the fat to use as the vital supply of energy.

For most people, it will only take 2-3 days to enter a state of ketosis. However, this will only happen if you are within your net carbs limit. It is much harder for people to shift into keto-adaption. Most adaptions will need to occur in the tissue, the brain, liver, kidney, and then the muscles. For some, it could take 3-4 weeks to use the ketones efficiently. This is the reason why it is important to stick with the diet to reap the benefits.

Getting into Keto-adaption

If you are looking to get into this as easily as possible, there are a few tricks you can do to facilitate the process:

1. Deplete Glycogen Quicker

2. Some studies have shown that all it takes is 1-2 exercise sessions to deplete the muscle glycogen. When this happens, it forces the body to use DNA and RNA to produce different compounds to fuel your body. If you deplete your body quicker, your body will turn to other fuel sources more quickly.

3. Increase Fat, Decrease Calories

   Generally, this isn't suggested. This is for those who want to get into the state of ketosis quicker. As you start your adaption process, you will want to ramp the exercise up and lower your calories. You will want to stabilize your body through eating enough healthy fats, so you are eating enough but also exercising more.

4. Protein Levels

   As you know, you will be eating a lot of healthy fat on this diet. Don't forget about the protein! Your body is going to be searching for the carbohydrates, and it can break down proteins into glucose. Remember that you want to use the fat as fuel. Be sure to always keep your protein levels in check. They should be consumed in moderation.

5. It will take time

   No matter what you try, the adaption will take time. You will eventually get to where you want to be, but you do not want to put your health at risk because you are trying too hard. Remember you've spent years running on glucose, it will take time for your body to adapt to ketosis. There are three phases you will be going through:

   a. Induction Phase

      Most weight loss during this phase will come from water weight loss.

b. Post-induction Stall Syndrome

This is when the balance of water and glycogen becomes set. This may stall your weight loss or can cause weight gain. Do not panic. Remember that this is part of the process and it is just water.

c. Keto-adaption

Conclusion

If you take anything away from this book, we ask you to be kind to yourself. Being on a new diet can be frustrating, intimidating, and terrifying. We are here to tell you that it doesn't have to be! Remember that you are doing this to benefit yourself, not torture yourself! As you know well, this process isn't easy. If you find yourself failing, remember that it is normal. It is something that everyone goes through. All you need to do is remind yourself that you have spent years developing your health habits. These aren't going to be erased over time. It will take some effort, but it will be worth it.

We hope that you can read this book and then take a good, hard look at your life choices. There has to be at least a reason that you are either A) not losing weight or B) gaining weight. Your body doesn't magically put on weight because it is plotting against your hard work. You may be working hard, but even one mistake can take away all your progress. So, which could it be? Are you miscounting your calories? Are you not measuring your ketones correctly? In the first few chapters, we offered a few different solutions to some of these issues. But remember, it could go deeper.

Let go of that obsession with your scale! There is no reason to fear being fat or becoming fat. If you are working hard, this is not something you need to be worried about. Through healthy life choices, that number on the scale will drop, we promise. You must promise yourself that you will stop obsessing over the number. Remember that the number in front of you does not determine the type of person you are or label you as a failure. If you are working as hard as you should be, it will drop in no time.

Now that you have gone through the process, it is time to continue your way down the path of the Ketogenic diet. You now know the basics of the diet and some mistakes you could be making. It is important that you realize your mistakes and try your best to correct them. Yes, you may trip and fall along the way, but what is important is that you get back up again. Never let anyone stand in your way of your goals, especially yourself. You deserve to be healthy and be happy. Remember that.